The Comprehensive Vegetarian Savory & Sweet Cookbook

Easy Savory And Sweet Vegetarian Recipes For Everyone

Adam Denton

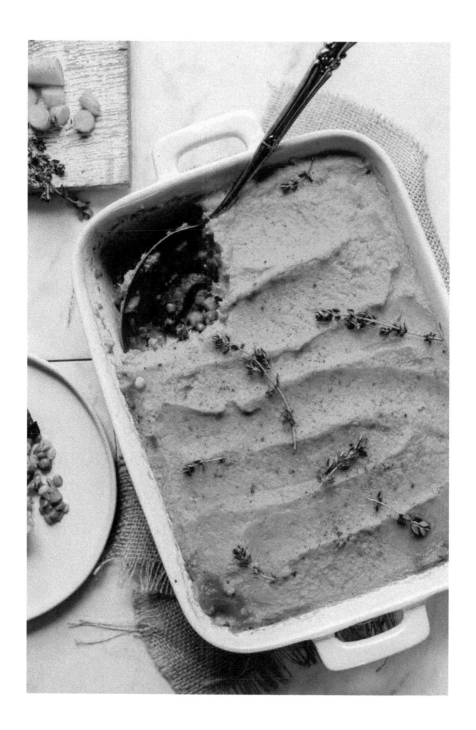

Table of contents

4

5

Reindeer food

Prep: 15 mins

Cook: 40 mins

Easy

Serves 6

Ingredients

- 150g porridge oats
- 150g jumbo oats
- 50g mixed nuts
- 25g pumpkin seeds
- 25g sunflower seeds
- 50g golden caster sugar
- 4 tbsp sunflower oil
- 2 tbsp maple syrup
- ½ tsp ground cinnamon
- ½ tsp mixed spice
- ½ tsp ground ginger
- 100g sultanas
- 100g apricots, chopped

• mixture of sweets (we used silver balls, chocolate beans, jelly sweets and hundreds and thousands)

Directions:

1 Heat oven to 140C/120C fan/gas

1. Put all the ingredients (except the apricots, sultanas and sweets) in a large bowl. Stir everything well, then spread out onto two baking trays in an even layer. Put the tray in the oven for 40 mins.

2. 2 Leave the granola to cool on the tray, then break it up into small chunks and stir in the sultanas and apricots.

3. Put the granola in a jar ready for breakfast. To make it suitable for magic reindeer, put a few spoonfuls into a small paper bag and mix in some sweets.

4. Tie with string or a ribbon and add a fun label for Father

Mini top-your-own pizzas

Prep: 1 hr and 25 mins

Cook:20 minsplus 1 hr 15 mins rising and proving

Easy

Makes 6

Ingredients

For the pizza base

- 300g strong white bread flour, plus extra for kneading
- 1 tbsp fast-action dried yeast
- 1 tsp caster sugar
- 1 tbsp olive oil, plus a little extra for greasing the bowl

For the pizza sauce

- 150ml passata
- small pack basil, leaves picked and finely chopped
- 1 tsp mixed herbs

For the toppings

- choose your favourites (we used black olives, yellow peppers, salami and grated cheddar)
- 200g ball mozzarella, torn into small pieces

Directions:

1. Put the flour in a large bowl. Add a little salt to one side of the bowl and the yeast to the other side. Sprinkle over the sugar, together with a spoon, and add the oil and 190ml warm water. Combine with a spoon until all the flour comes away from the sides of the bowl, then tip onto a floured surface. Knead for 5-10 mins or until smooth and elastic. Lightly oil a clean bowl, add the dough, cover with cling film and leave to rise for 1 hr.

2. Meanwhile, make the sauce. Pour the passata into a saucepan, add the basil and mixed herbs, then season and bring to the boil over a low heat. Simmer gently for 5 mins, then set aside to cool. Chop the toppings.

3. Once the dough has risen, tip it out, knock out the air and divide into 6 equal parts. Heat oven to 240C/220C fan/gas 9 and place 2 large baking sheets in the oven.

4. Roll out the dough on a lightly floured surface into a circle around 15cm in diameter. Pick up the circle of dough and toss about a metre up, spinning it in the air. Catch it on the back of your hand, so your fingers don't poke through the dough. Do this at least 3 times to achieve a thin central base and a thicker outside crust. Alternatively, you could carry on rolling, but it's not as much fun!

5. Lay the bases onto baking parchment (2 bases on 1 piece of parchment) and carefully slide each pair inside a plastic bag 'tent' for 15 mins to prove again.

6. After the second rise, spread the sauce over the bases and add the and mozzarella. Take the baking sheets out the oven and quickly slide the pizzas (still on their baking parchment) on top. You can cook 2-3 pizzas per tray. Return to the oven and bake for 12 mins. Take out, slice and eat.

Caramel & coffee ice cream sandwich

Prep: 5 mins, plus at least a few hours freezing, no cook

Easy

Serves 2

Ingredients

- 1 tbsp chocolate-coated coffee beans, roughly chopped
- 2 scoops coffee ice cream, softened
- 4 caramel wafers

Directions:

1. Mix the chocolate coffee beans into the softened ice cream until combined, then transfer to a small loaf tin and freeze for a few hours or until solid.

2. Use cookie cutters to cut the ice cream to the same size as the waffles, then sandwich between two waffles.

Eyeball snot-tail

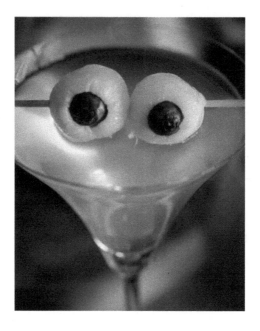

Prep: 25 mins plus chilling, no cook

Easy

Serves 10 – 15

Ingredients
• 135g pack lime jelly
• 700ml apple & pear juice (we used Copella)
• 300ml lemonade

- 425g can lychees in syrup
- 10-15 cocktail cherries from a jar
- 10-15 raisins You will need
- 10-15 cocktail sticks

Directions:

1. Make the jelly following pack instructions and chill until set. Combine the apple & pear juice with the lemonade in a large jug and chill in the fridge.

2. To make the eyeballs, drain the lychees and poke a hole in each cherry with one of the cocktail sticks. Put the cherry inside the lychee, then push the raisin into the cherry. Press the eyeball onto the end of a cocktail stick and set aside until serving.

3. When the jelly has set, use a whisk to break it up into small chunks. Spoon into the cocktail glasses and top up with the apple juice mixture. Put an eyeball into each glass before serving.

Christmas tree pops

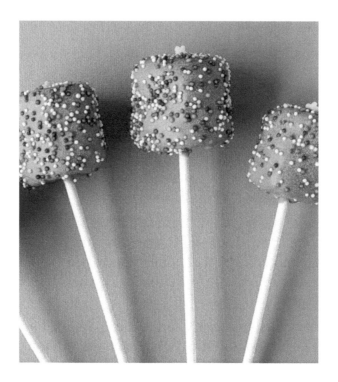

Prep: 1 hr

Cook: 20 mins plus setting

Easy

Makes 8

Ingredients

- 100g butter at room temperature, plus extra for greasing
- 100g golden caster sugar
- 1 tsp vanilla extract
- 2 medium eggs
- 100g self-raising flour
- 3 tbsp cocoa powder
- 3 tbsp milk
- 300g icing sugar, sifted
- green food colouring
- sprinkles, for decorating (we used sugar snowflakes and mini Smarties)
- 8 lollipops or cake pop sticks, to serve

Directions:

1. Heat oven to 180C/160C fan/gas 4. Grease a 20cm round cake tin and line the base with a circle of baking parchment.

2. Put the butter in a big mixing bowl with the sugar and vanilla extract, and mix until it looks creamy. Crack in the eggs, one at a time, mixing after each one. Sift the flour and cocoa together, add to the bowl with the milk and stir everything together until smooth. Spoon into the cake tin and use the back of a wooden spoon to spread the top to make it as flat as you can. Bake for 20 mins until a skewer poked into the centre comes out clean, with just cake crumbs stuck to it, not wet batter. Leave the cake to cool completely in the tin on a wire rack.

3. Remove the cake from the tin and use a serrated knife to cut it into 8 wedges. Turn each one so that the round, outside edge is facing you, and push a lollipop or cake pop stick through the middle of the outside edge. Remember to leave enough of the stick poking out for you to hold.

4. Mix the food colouring and icing sugar with enough water to make an icing that is a bit runny, but still quite stiff. Try drizzling a bit on a spare piece of paper; you want it to stay in strips, not run all over the place.

5. Spoon some icing over each cake wedge (you can cover it completely or drizzle lines across them in a tree shape). Decorate with sugar snowflakes and mini Smarties, then lift onto a wire rack and leave to set completely (this will take a few hours). Iced cakes will keep in the tin for up to 2 days. The un-iced cake can be frozen for up to 6 months. Defrost completely before cutting and decorating.

Sweet & sticky wings with classic slaw

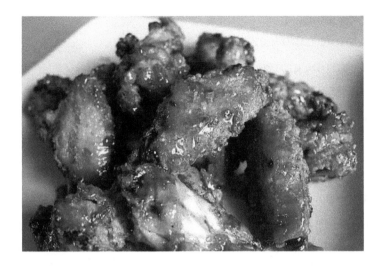

Prep: 10 mins

Cook:40 mins

Easy

Serves 6

Ingredients
- 4 tbsp ketchup
- 4 garlic cloves, crushed
- 3 tbsp soft brown sugar

- 4 tbsp sweet chilli sauce
- 4 tbsp dark soy sauce
- 1kg chicken wings
- 1 small white cabbage, shredded
- 3 large carrots, grated
- 1 large onion, thinly sliced
- 8 tbsp light salad cream or mayonnaise

Directions:

1. Heat oven to 200C/180C fan/gas 6. In a large bowl, mix the ketchup, garlic, sugar, half the sweet chilli sauce and the soy sauce with some seasoning. Tip in the wings and toss to combine so that they are all coated. Transfer to a large roasting tray or two smaller ones, in a single layer. Roast for 35-40 mins until cooked through and golden.

2. Meanwhile, make the slaw. Mix the vegetables with remaining chilli sauce, salad cream or mayo and seasoning. Pile the wings onto a large platter and transfer the slaw to a serving bowl. Let everyone dig in and help themselves.

Icy kir

Prep:5 mins

No cook

Easy

Serves 1

Ingredients

- 25ml vodka
- a scoop of blackcurrant or raspberry sorbet
- 100ml prosecco

Directions:

Pour the vodka into the bottom of a coupe glass. Chill for 30 mins, then top with the blackcurrant or raspberry sorbet and pour the Prosecco around it. Serve immediately.

Milkshake ice pops

Prep:10 mins plus 4 hrs freezing

No cook

Easy

Makes 4

Ingredients

- 405ml can light condensed milk
- 1 tsp vanilla bean paste
- 1 ripe chopped banana
- 10 strawberries or 3 tbsp chocolate hazelnut spread

Directions:

1. Pour the light condensed milk into a food processor and add the vanilla bean paste and chopped banana. Whizz until smooth. Add either the strawberries or chocolate hazelnut spread and whizz again.

2. Divide the mixture between 4 paper cups, cover with foil, then push a lolly stick through the foil lid of each cup until you hit the base. Freeze for 4 hrs or until solid. Will keep in the freezer for 2 months.

Breakfast bar

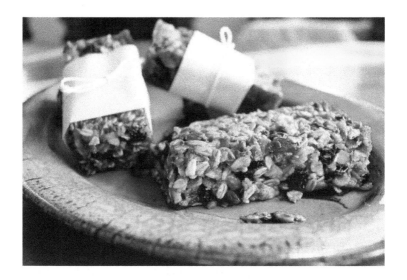

Prep:20 mins

Cook:25 mins

Easy

Makes 12

Ingredients

• 50g mixed dried fruit (a mixture of raisins, sultanas and apricots is nice)

• 50g mixed seed

- 140g oats
- 25g multi-grain hoop cereal
- 100g butter
- 100g light muscovado sugar
- 100g golden syrup

Directions:

1. Grease and line a 20cm square cake tin with baking parchment.

2. Put the dried fruit in a mixing bowl. Add the seeds, oats and cereal, and mix well.

3. Put the butter, sugar and golden syrup in the saucepan. Cook gently on the hob, stirring with the spatula, until the butter and sugar are melted. Remove from the heat and pour the dry Ingredients into the saucepan.

4. Mix well until all the Ingredients are coated with the syrup mix.

5. Fill the baking tin with the mixture. Use the spatula to press the mix down evenly. Bake at 160C/140C fan/gas 3 for 20 mins, then leave to cool completely before cutting into squares or fingers. Store in an airtight tin for up to 3 days– if they last that long!

Crispy chocolate fridge cake

Prep:15 mins

Cook:5 mins Plus chilling

Easy

Makes 16-20 chunks

Ingredients

- 300g dark chocolate, broken into chunks
- 100g butter, diced
- 140g golden syrup
- 1 tsp vanilla extract
- 200g biscuit, roughly chopped
- 100g sultana
- 85g Rice Krispies
- 100-140g mini eggs (optional)
- 50g white chocolate, melted

Directions:

1. Line a 20 x 30cm tin with baking parchment. Melt the chocolate, butter and golden syrup in a bowl set over a pan of simmering water, stirring occasionally, until smooth

and glossy. Add the vanilla, biscuits, sultanas and Rice Krispies, and mix well until everything is coated.

2. Tip the mixture into the tin, then flatten it down with the back of a spoon. Press in some mini eggs, if using, and put in the fridge until set. When hard, drizzle all over with the melted white chocolate and set again before cutting into chunks.

Pea hummus

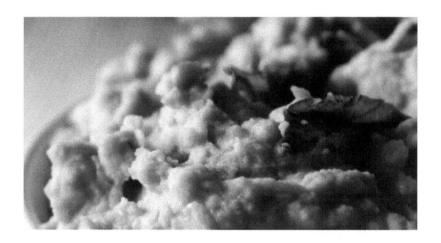

Prep: 10 mins

No cook

Easy

Serves 4

Ingredients
- 200g cooked peas
- 1 garlic clove, crushed
- 1 tbsp tahini
- squeeze of lemon

- 1 tbsp cooked cannellini beans, from a can
- 2 tbsp olive oil
- strips of pitta bread, to serve
- raw vegetable sticks, to serve

Directions:

Blitz all the Ingredients together using a hand blender or food processor. Add 1-2 tbsp water, then blitz again. Transfer a portion to a pot and add to a lunchbox with pitta bread strips and veg sticks. Keep the rest chilled for up to 3 days.

Lemon curd & blueberry loaf cake

Prep: 20 mins

Cook: 1 hr and 15 mins

Easy

Cuts into 8-10 slices

Ingredients

• 175g softened butter, plus extra for greasing
• 500ml tub Greek yogurt (you need 100ml/3.5fl oz in the cake, the rest to serve)
• 300g jar good lemon curd (you need 2 tbsp in the cake, the rest to serve)
• 3 eggs
• zest and juice 1 lemon, plus extra zest to serve, if you like
• 200g self-raising flour
• 175g golden caster sugar
• 200g punnet of blueberries (you need 85g/3oz in the cake, the rest to serve)
• 140g icing sugar
• edible flowers, such as purple or yellow primroses, to serve (optional)

Directions:

1. Heat oven to 160C/140C fan/gas 3. Grease a 2lb loaf tin and line with a long strip of baking parchment. Put 100g yogurt, 2 tbsp lemon curd, the softened butter, eggs, lemon zest, flour and caster sugar into a large mixing bowl. Quickly mix with an electric whisk until the batter just comes together. Scrape half into the prepared tin. Weigh 85g blueberries from the punnet and sprinkle half into the tin, scrape the rest of the batter on top, then scatter the other half of the 85g berries on top. Bake for 1 hr 10 mins-1 hr 15 mins until golden, and a skewer poked into the centre comes out clean.

2. Cool in the tin, then carefully lift onto a serving plate to ice. Sift the icing sugar into a bowl and stir in enough lemon juice to make a thick, smooth icing. Spread over the top of the cake, then decorate with lemon zest and edible flowers, if you like. Serve in slices with extra lemon curd, Greek yogurt and blueberries.

Easy lamb tagine

Prep: 10 mins

Cook: 2 hrs and 10 mins

Easy

Serves a family of 4-6 or makes 6-8 toddler meals

Ingredients

- 2 tbsp olive oil
- 1 onion, finely diced
- 2 carrots, finely diced (about 150g)
- 500g diced leg of lamb
- 2 fat cloves garlic, crushed
- ½ tsp cumin
- ½ tsp ground ginger
- ¼ tsp saffron strands
- 1 tsp ground cinnamon
- 1 tbsp clear honey
- 100g soft dried apricot, quartered
- 1 low-salt vegetable stock cube
- 1 small butternut squash, peeled, seeds removed and cut into 1cm dice

- steamed couscous or rice, to serve
- chopped parsley and toasted pine nuts, to serve (optional)

Directions:

1. Heat the olive oil in a heavy-based pan and add the onion and carrot. Cook for 3- 4 mins until softened.

2. Add the diced lamb and brown all over. Stir in the garlic and all the spices and cook for a few mins more or until the aromas are released.

3. Add the honey and apricots, crumble in the stock cube and pour over roughly 500ml boiling water or enough to cover the meat. Give it a good stir and bring to the boil. Turn down to a simmer, put the lid on and cook for 1 hour.

4. Remove the lid and cook for a further 30 mins, then stir in the squash. Cook for 20 – 30 mins more until the squash is soft and the lamb is tender. Serve alongside rice or couscous and sprinkle with parsley and pine nuts, if using.

Bread in four easy

Prep: 15 mins

Cook: 35 mins Plus rising

Easy

Cuts into 8 thick slices

Ingredients

• 500g granary, strong wholewheat or white bread flour (I used granary)
• 7g sachet fast-action dried yeast
• 1 tsp salt
• 2 tbsp olive oil
• 1 tbsp clear honey

Directions:

1. Tip the flour, yeast and salt into a large bowl and mix together with your hands. Stir 300ml handhot water with the oil and honey, then stir into the dry Ingredients to make a soft dough.

2. Turn the dough out onto a lightly floured surface and knead for 5 mins, until the dough no longer feels sticky, sprinkling with a little more flour if you need it.

3. Oil a 900g loaf tin and put the dough in the tin, pressing it in evenly.

4. Put in a large plastic food bag and leave to rise for 1 hr, until the dough has risen to fill the tin and it no longer springs back when you press it with your finger.

5. Heat oven to 200C/fan 180C/gas

6. Make several slashes across the top of the loaf with a sharp knife, then bake for 30-35 mins until the loaf is risen and golden. Tip it out onto a cooling rack and tap the base of the bread to check it is cooked. It should sound hollow. Leave to cool.

Bespoke martini kit Easy

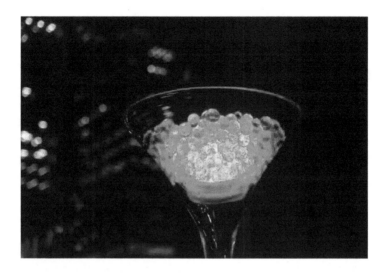

Ingredients

- 700ml bottle rye vodka
- small pot of juniper berries
- small pod of green cardamom pods
- small pot of dried rose petals
- small pot of coriander seeds
- 1 lemon
- 1 coffee filter paper
- bottle of vermouth
- small jar of green olives Optional extras
- 2 martini glasses
- shot measure
- tall glass

- cocktail stirrer
- cocktail strainer

Directions:

1. To use the kit: Write the following instructions on the gift tag: Open the bottle of vodka and add 2 tbsp juniper berries, 6 cardamom pods, a pinch of dried rose petals, 1 tsp coriander seeds and a strip of lemon peel. Put the lid back on and leave in a cool dark place for 24 hrs.

2. Strain the infused mixture through the coffee filter paper into a jug, then pour back into the bottle to store.

3. To make a martini, chill 2 martini glasses in the fridge for 30 mins. Put 50ml vermouth in a tall glass, add 150ml infused vodka and a large handful of ice. Stir well until the outside of the glass feels cold, then strain into the chilled glasses. Garnish with an olive.

Sausage plait

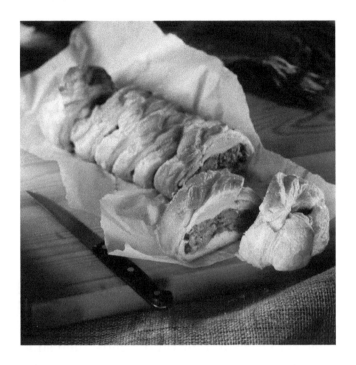

Prep:30 mins

Cook:40 mins

Easy

Serves 4

Ingredients

- a little oil, for greasing
- 400g pack pork and apple sausage - about 6 fat sausages
- 1 roasted red pepper from a jar, patted dry with kitchen paper
- 1 large egg
- ½ tsp chilli flakes (optional)
- 2 tbsp tomato purée
- flour, for dusting
- 250g ready-made puff pastry
- baked beans or salad, to serve

Directions:

1. Heat oven to 200C/180C fan/ gas 6. Grease a baking tray with oil using a pastry brush, then cover it with baking parchment. Put to one side. Remove the meat from the sausage skins by snipping off the ends, then squeezing the sausagemeat into a bowl (see 1).Cut the pepper into small pieces with scissors. Break the egg into the cup, beat with a fork, and save 2 tbsp for glazing. Add the red pepper and remaining egg to the sausagemeat with the chilli flakes, if using, and purée.

2. Mix well with a fork or clean hands

3. Sprinkle some flour on the work surface. Using a rolling pin, roll out the pastry into a rough square shape, about 30 x 30cm. Put the pastry on the lined baking tray (3).

4. Now spoon the filling down the middle of the pastry in a sausage shape – leave a little gap at the top and bottom (about 3cm) (4).

5. Cut the pastry at a slight diagonal, on either side of the filling, into 1.5cm strips, the same number each side– we

cut 12 strips each side. Brush the pastry all over with most of the saved egg (5).

6. Tuck the top and bottom edges of the pastry over the filling. Starting at the top, lay the pastry strips over the filling, taking one from each side, to cross like a plait. Now brush the top all over with the last of the egg. Bake for 35-40 mins or until golden. Serve hot or cold with baked beans or salad (6).

Blackberry & apple loaf

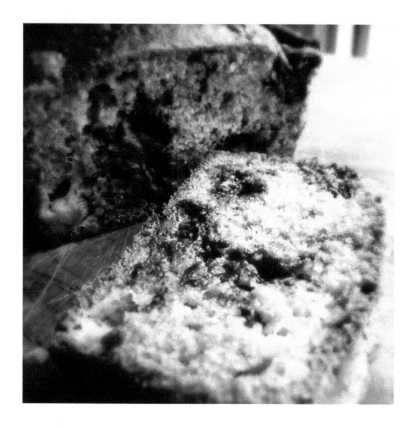

Total time: 2 hrs

Ready in 2 hours, including baking

Easy

Cuts into 10 chunky slices

Ingredients

- 250g self-raising flour
- 175g butter
- 175g light muscovado sugar
- ½ tsp cinnamon
- 2rounded tbsp demerara sugar
- 1 small eating apple,such as Cox's, quartered (not cored or peeled)
- 2 large eggs, beaten
- 1 orange, finely grated zest
- 1 tsp baking powder
- 225g blackberry

Directions:

1. Preheat the oven to 180C/gas 4/fan 160C. Butter and line the bottom of a 1.7 litre loaf tin (see tip below). In a large bowl, rub the flour, butter and muscovado sugar together with your fingers to make fine crumbs. Measure out 5 level tbsp of this mixture into a small bowl for the topping, and mix in to it the cinnamon and demerara sugar. Set aside.

2. Coarsely grate the apple down to the core and mix in with the eggs and the zest. Stir the baking powder into the rubbed-in mixture in the large bowl, then quickly and lightly stir in the egg mixture until it drops lightly from the spoon. Don't overmix.

3. Gently fold in three quarters of the berries with a metal spoon, trying not to break them up. Spoon into the tin and

level. Scatter the rest of the berries on top. Sprinkle over the topping and bake for 1¼ -1 hour 20 minutes. Check after 50 minutes and cover loosely with foil if it is browning too much. When done the cake will feel firm, but test with a skewer.

4. Leave in the tin for 30 minutes before turning out, then cool on a wire rack. Peel off the paper before cutting. Will keep wrapped in foil or in a tin for up to 2 days

Chocolate marble pancakes

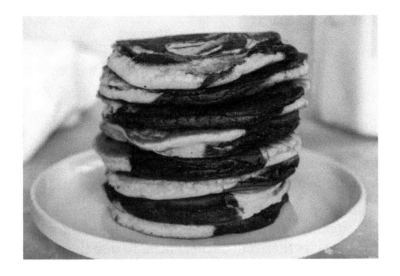

Prep:10 mins

Cook:10 mins

Easy makes 12

Ingredients
• 200g self-raising flour
• 2 eggs
• 2 tbsp caster sugar
• 300ml whole milk
• 1 tsp vanilla extract

- 2 tbsp cocoa powder
- oil for frying
- chocolate sauce, to serve

Directions:

1. Put the flour, eggs and sugar into a bowl. Pour in the milk and whisk until you have a smooth batter, then divide in half. To one half of the batter, whisk in the vanilla extract, and to the other half, whisk in the cocoa powder.

2. Lightly oil a non-stick pan, set over a medium heat. Using two spoons, alternately drop the white and dark batter on top of each other, a little off centre, so that the colours very slightly spread until you have 4 concentric circles. Cook until the underside is bubbly then flip and cook for 30 seconds more. Repeat the process with the rest of the batter. Serve drizzled with chocolate sauce.

Sweet sushi

Prep:40 mins

Cook:5 mins plus setting

Easy

Makes 24

Ingredients

• 45g butter
• 280g marshmallows
• 340g Rice Krispies To decorate
• 10 cola belts
• 50g dark or milk chocolate, melted
• 50g millions
• 50g apricot jam
• 2 red pencil sweets
• 2 green pencil sweets
• 100g ready-to-roll fondant icing
• orange, red and purple food colouring
• white and green food colouring powder
• 25g black treacle

Directions:

1. To make your bases melt the butter and marshmallows in a large saucepan. Once melted, gently stir in the Rice Krispies.

2. Pour the mixture onto a lined 30cm x 20cm tray and press down firmly to compact the Rice Krispies and make flat. Leave to set for 1-2 hours. Once set, cut out 12 small circles with a small round cutter using a small sharp knife to cut all the way through to the bottom if needed. Use the rest of the mix to make 10 rectangular pieces.

3. Cut your cola belts to size, measuring them around the cutter. Stick them with a small smudge of melted chocolate. Repeat on all 10 and leave to set. Mix the millions and jam together and put small heaps on 6 of the circles to look like caviar. On the remaining 6 pieces, get a chopstick and make 4 indents in the centre of the rice. Cut your pencil sweets into small pieces and poke them into the indents alternating in colour.

4. To decorate the rectangles, split your fondant icing in half and colour half orange and half a purple/red colour so they look like salmon and tuna. Roll each out to 5mm thick. Use a knife to cut out shapes that will fit on top of the rectangles and use the back of a knife to make fine imprints to make the pieces more flesh-like. On the orange 'salmon' pieces, paint the imprints with the white colouring powder. Place all the bits of decorated icing on top of the rectangular bases, moulding them to look as natural as possible.

5. Use the green food colouring powder to brush the cola belts and create a seaweed effect.

6. Finally to make your 'soy sauce' heat the black treacle and 50ml water in a pan until combined. Brush over the 'tuna' and 'salmon' sushi pieces and put the rest in a bowl as a dipping sauce.

Barbecued chicken fajita skewers

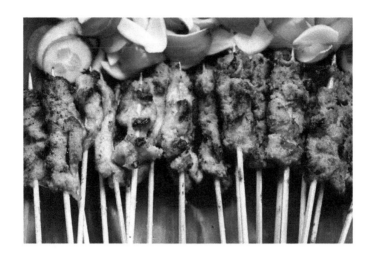

Prep:30 mins

Cook:10 mins

Easy

Makes 6-8 skewers

Ingredients

For the fajitas

• 2 limes, plus wedges to serve

• 1 tsp dried oregano

• 1 tsp ground cumin

- 1 tsp smoked paprika
- 1 tsp olive oil
- 2 garlic cloves, crushed or finely grated
- 4 chicken breasts
- 3 mixed coloured peppers
- 1 red onion for the guacamole
- 2 ripe avocados
- 1 lime
- 6 cherry tomatoes, halved
- warmed tortillas, chopped coriander, soured cream or yogurt, plus chilli sauce for the grownups, to serve

Directions:

1. Make the marinade. In a large bowl, juice both the limes. Add the oregano, spices, olive oil and garlic, and mix together. Dice the chicken, then get your child to stir it through the marinade, and set aside.

2. Prepare the vegetables. Deseeding the peppers and halving the onion is tricky, so do this yourself. Children aged from about seven or above can cut them into chunks using a child-friendly knife.

3. Make your skewers. Carefully thread alternate pieces of chicken, peppers and onion onto your skewers. Smaller children might find this a little hard, so the best way is to stab the Ingredients and push them up the skewers. When you've used up all the Ingredients, set aside. Can be made several hours ahead and chilled until ready to cook.

4. Prepare the guacamole. Stone and peel the avocados, then tip into a bowl with the other Ingredients. Get your child

to use a potato masher to mash everything together and tip into a serving dish.

5. Cook the skewers. Heat a barbecue or griddle pan. Cook the skewers for 10-12 mins, turning, until they are cooked all the way through. A child from the age of eight can watch over a griddle and turn the skewers with a pair of tongs. Serve the skewers on heated tortillas with the guacamole, soured cream, chopped coriander, lime wedges on the side and chilli sauce for those who like a touch of spice.

Winter wonderland cake

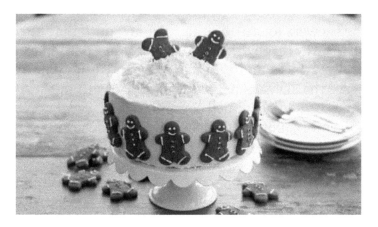

Prep:1 hr

Cook:35 mins Plus cooling

Easy

Serves 12

Ingredients
- 175g unsalted butter, softened, plus more for the tin
- 250g golden caster sugar
- 3 large eggs
- 225g plain flour
- 2 tsp baking powder
- 50g crème fraîche

- 100g dark chocolate, melted and cooled a little
- 3 tbsp strawberry jam
- 8-10 candy canes, red and white
- mini white meringues and jelly sweets, to decorate For the angel frosting
- 500g white caster sugar
- 1 tsp vanilla extract
- 1 tbsp liquid glucose
- 2 egg whites
- 30g icing sugar, sifted

Directions:

1. Heat oven to 180C/160C fan/gas 4. Butter and line three 18cm (or two 20cm) cake tins. Beat the butter and sugar together until light and fluffy. Add the eggs, beating them in one at a time. Fold in the flour, baking powder and a pinch of salt, then fold in the crème fraîche and chocolate and 100ml boiling water.

2. Divide the cake mixture between the tins and level the tops of the batter. Bake for 25-30 mins or until a skewer inserted into the middle comes out clean. Leave to cool for 10 mins in the tin, then tip out onto a cooling rack and peel off the parchment. Set aside to cool completely.

3. To make the angel frosting, put the sugar, vanilla and liquid glucose in a pan with 125ml water. Bring to the boil and cook until the sugar has melted – the syrup turns clear and the mixture hits 130C on a sugar thermometer (be very careful with hot sugar). Take off the heat. Meanwhile, beat the egg whites until stiff then, while still beating, gradually pour in the hot sugar syrup in a steady stream. Keep

49

beating until the mixture is fluffy and thick enough to spread – this might take a few mins as the mixture cools. Beat in the icing sugar.

4. Spread two of the sponges with jam and some of the icing mixture, then sandwich the cakes together with the plain one on top. Use a little of the frosting to ice the whole cake (don't worry about crumbs at this stage). Use the remaining icing to ice the cake again, smoothing the side, and swirling it on top. Crush four of the candy canes and sprinkle over the cake, then add the remaining whole candy canes, meringues and sweets.

Nutty cinnamon & yogurt dipper

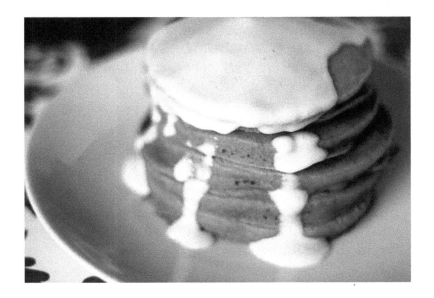

Prep:5 mins

No cook

Easy Serves 1

Ingredients

- 100g natural Greek yogurt
- 1 tbsp nut butter (try almond or cashew)
- ¼ tsp ground cinnamon
- 1 tsp honey To serve

- apple wedges (tossed in a little lemon juice to prevent them turning brown)

- celery sticks

- carrot sticks

- mini rice cakes or crackers (choose gluten-free brands if necessary)

Directions:

In a small tub, mix together the yogurt, nut butter, cinnamon and honey. Serve with apple wedges (tossed in a little lemon juice to prevent them turning brown), celery or carrot sticks, and mini rice cakes or crackers.

Pressed picnic sandwich

Prep:25 mins

Cook:3 mins

Easy

Serves 8

Ingredients

- long ciabatta loaf, sliced in half lengthways
- 3 tbsp olive oil
- 1 tbsp balsamic vinegar
- 2 garlic cloves, finely chopped
- 1 tsp Dijon mustard
- 2 big handfuls of baby spinach
- 8 marinated artichoke hearts from a jar, quartered
- 250g roasted red pepper from a jar
- 8 slices prosciutto
- big handful of basil
- 125g ball mozzarella, cut into slices
- ½ red onion, very finely sliced

Directions:

1. Ask an adult to slice the ciabatta loaf in half lengthways and heat the oven to 200C/180C fan/gas 6.

2. Put the ciabatta loaf halves, crust-side down, on a large baking tray and drizzle with a little olive oil. Pop them in the oven for a few mins until just golden and lightly toasted.

3. Put the olive oil, balsamic vinegar, garlic and mustard in a bowl, then whisk them together with a fork.

4. Remove the toasted ciabatta halves from the tray and drizzle the bottom slice with about half of the dressing.

5. Arrange the rest of the Ingredients in layers. Start with a large handful of baby spinach, then a few artichoke hearts.

6. Next add the slices of pepper, the prosciutto, basil, mozzarella and, finally, the red onion.

7. Drizzle over the rest of the dressing and pop the other slice of ciabatta on top.

8. Press down on the sandwich to squash all the layers together.

9. Wrap the sandwich in baking parchment and tie it together with a couple of pieces of string.

10. Place a heavy baking tray on top of your sandwich and top it with weights or loaf tins filled with baking beans. Pop it all in the fridge overnight or until you are ready to eat it. Cut and serve in slices for the perfect picnic snack.

Whisky & pink peppercorn marmalade kit Easy

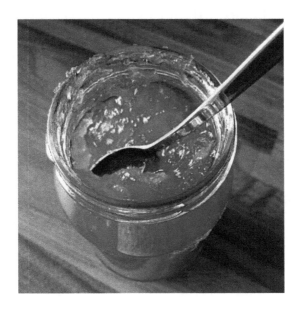

Ingredients

- 500g mix of oranges, clementines and lemons
- 1kg demerara sugar
- small pot of pink peppercorns
- small bottle of whisky Optional extras
- jam pan muslin
- large wooden spoon
- small jars and labels (makes about 1kg jam)

To use kit see tip

Directions:

<u>To use the kit:</u>

1. Write the following instructions on the gift tag:Halve the fruits and squeeze the juices into a large saucepan. Remove all the peel and set aside. Put the flesh in the pan with 1 litre water and boil for 15 mins. Push through a sieve lined with muslin and return the liquid to the pan.

2. Shred the peel and tip into a heatproof bowl. Add enough water to just cover and microwave for 3-4 mins until soft. Add the peel to the pan, then add the sugar. Boil for 35-45 mins until the marmalade has reached setting point (keep an eye on it so it doesn't bubble over).

3. Remove from the heat and add 1 tsp pink peppercorns. Allow the mixture to cool a little, then stir in 50ml whisky. Ladle into sterilised jars and seal. Will keep for up to one year.

Coconut bauble truffles

Prep:45 mins plus at least 2 hrs chilling,

No Cook

Easy

Makes about 20

Ingredients

• 250g madeira cake

• 85g ready-to-eat dried apricots, finely chopped
• 25g desiccated coconut

• 125ml light condensed milk To decorate

• 140g desiccated coconut

• different food colourings, we used yellow, pink, blue and purple

Directions:

1. In a big mixing bowl, crumble the cake with your fingers – try to get the bits as small as possible.

2. Tip in the apricots and coconut. Using your hands again, mix together with the cake crumbs. Use a wooden spoon to stir in the condensed milk. After you've mixed it in a bit,

use your fingers to pull off any bits stuck to the spoon. Squidge everything together with your hands until it is well mixed and all the cake crumbs are sticky. Rub your hands together over the bowl so any bits that are stuck drop off.

3. Line some trays that fit in your fridge with baking parchment. Roll the sticky cake mixture into small balls (about the size of a conker or gobstopper) between your hands. Line them up on the trays, then put them in the fridge while you get the decorations ready.

4. Decide on how many different food colourings you are going to use, then split the coconut into the same number of piles. Put each pile of coconut into a plastic sandwich bag, add a few drops of food colouring to each, and tie a knot in the top. Shake the bags and scrunch between your fingers until all the coconut is coloured – if it's not bright enough, open the bag and add a few more drops of colouring.

5. Open all the bags of coloured coconut and take the truffles from the fridge. Put 1 tbsp of water in a small bowl and lightly coat each truffle in it so the coconut can stick to the outside of each bauble.

6. One by one, drop each truffle into one of your bags. Shake it and roll it around until the outside is covered in coconut. Carefully put each truffle back onto the trays and chill for at least another 2 hrs until they are really cold and firm.

7. If you like, put some of the truffles in gift bags or boxes and tie with ribbons to give as presents. Will keep in the fridge for up to 1 week.

Best ever pesto & potato pasta

Prep:20 mins

Cook:11 mins

Easy

Serves 4 - 6

Ingredients

• 150g green bean

• 300g new potato

• 300g short dried pasta like fusilli or a long pasta like linguine

• For the pesto

• large bunch basil

• 50g pine nuts

• 50g parmesan (or vegetarian alternative), grated, plus extra to serve (optional)

• 2 garlic cloves

• 100ml olive oil

Directions:

1. <u>KIDS</u>: **the writing in bold is for you.** <u>GROWN-UPS</u>: the rest is for you. Pick the basil for the pesto. **Get your child to pick the basil leaves off the stalks. Ask them to look at and smell the leaves as you tell them the name of the herb until they remember it** – try to do this with all herbs when you can.

2. Make the pesto. Toast the pine nuts in a pan over a low heat. **A child of seven years plus can stir the nuts in the pan.** Tip into a mini chopper (or use a pestle and mortar) with the basil, parmesan, garlic and olive oil. Blitz or pound into a green sauce, then set aside.

3. Chop up the beans. **Using a child-friendly knife, get children from the age of five to chop the green beans into shorter lengths, and quarter the potatoes. Younger children can snap the beans into short lengths** while you prepare the potatoes.

4. Cook the vegetables and pasta. Bring a large pan of water to the boil, add the potatoes and boil for 3 mins. Remove from the heat and **ask the child to tip in the pasta and give it a stir.** Put the pan back on the heat, boil the pasta for 5 mins, add the beans and cook for a final 3 mins.

5. Mix everything together. Drain everything well and tip into a bowl. **Spoon most of the pesto into the pasta and stir everything together to coat.** Bring the large bowl of pasta to the table and serve with extra parmesan, more basil and remaining pesto, if you like.

Simnel muffins

Prep:45 mins - 55 mins

Easy

Makes 12

Ingredients
- 250g mixed dried fruit
- grated zest and juice 1 medium orange
- 175g softened butter
- 175g golden caster sugar
- 3 eggs, beaten
- 300g self-raising flour
- 1 tsp mixed spice
- ½ tsp freshly grated nutmeg
- 5 tbsp milk
- 175g marzipan
- 200g icing sugar
- 2 tbsp orange juice for mixing
- mini eggs

Directions:

1. Tip the fruit into a bowl, add the zest and juice and microwave on medium for 2 minutes (or leave to soak for 1 hour). Line 12 deep muffin tins with paper muffin cases.

2. Preheat the oven to fan 180C/ 160C/gas 4. Beat together the butter, sugar, eggs, flour, spices and milk until light and fluffy (about 3-5 minutes) – use a wooden spoon or hand held mixer. Stir the fruit in well.

3. Half fill the muffin cases with the mixture. Divide the marzipan into 12 equal pieces, roll into balls, then flatten with your thumb to the size of the muffin cases. Put one into each muffin case and spoon the rest of the mixture over it. Bake for 25-30 minutes, until risen, golden and firm to the touch. Leave to cool.

4. Beat together the icing sugar and orange juice to make icing thick enough to coat the back of a wooden spoon. Drizzle over the muffins and top with a cluster of eggs. Leave to set. Best eaten within a day of making.

Chicken schnitzel strips with tomato spaghetti

Prep:30 mins

Cook:20 mins

Easy

Serves 4

Ingredients
- 2 large eggs, beaten
- 3 tbsp plain flour
- 2 tbsp grated parmesan
- zest 1 lemon
- 150g fresh white breadcrumbs
- 4 small chicken breasts
- 350g spaghetti
- 3 tbsp sunflower oil
- rocket leaf or green salad, to serve For the tomato sauce
- 400g can chopped tomatoes with olive oil and garlic
- 1 tbsp tomato purée
- handful basil leaves, torn

63

Directions:

1. First, make the tomato sauce. Tip the tomatoes into a medium saucepan and add 1 /2 a can of water. Stir in the tomato purée, season and simmer for 15 mins. Keep warm while you make the chicken.

2. Put the eggs in a shallow dish. Lightly season the flour and tip it into another shallow dish. Mix the Parmesan, lemon zest and breadcrumbs together and tip onto a plate.

3. Place each chicken breast between two sheets of cling film on a chopping board. Ask your child to help bash them gently with a rolling pin until they are about 2cm thick. Cut each flattened chicken breast into five or six strips.

4. Cook the spaghetti in a pan of boiling salted water for 10-12 mins or following pack instructions. Get your child to help you coat the chicken strips in the flour and shake off any excess. Dip them in the beaten egg, letting any excess drip off, then finally coat them well in the breadcrumbs and put on a plate. Once all the chicken strips are coated, heat the oil in a large frying pan until hot.

5. Add the chicken strips to the pan in batches and fry for 2-3 mins each side until cooked through – you may need to wipe out the pan in between batches. Lift out and drain on kitchen paper.

6. Drain the spaghetti, then mix with the tomato sauce. Serve alongside the chicken strips and some rocket leaves or a crisp green salad.

Eerie eyeball pops

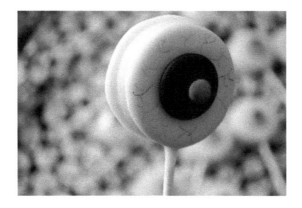

Prep: 30 mins

Cook: 5 mins plus chilling

Easy

Makes 10

Ingredients

- 100g/4oz madeira cake
- 100g Oreo cookie
- 100g bar milk chocolate, melted
- 200g bar white chocolate, melted
- few Smarties and icing pens, to decorate You will also need 10 wooden skewers

• ½ small pumpkin or butternut squash, deseeded, to stand pops in

Directions:

1. Break the Madeira cake and cookies into the bowl of a food processor, pour in the melted milk chocolate and whizz to combine.

2. Tip the mixture into a bowl, then use your hands to roll into about 10 walnut-sized balls. Chill for 2 hrs until really firm.

3. Push a skewer into each ball, then carefully spoon the white chocolate over the cake balls to completely cover. Stand the cake pops in the pumpkin, then press a Smartie onto the surface while wet. Chill again until the chocolate has set. Before serving, using the icing pens, add a pupil to each Smartie and wiggly red veins to the eyeballs.

Easy tuna pasta bake

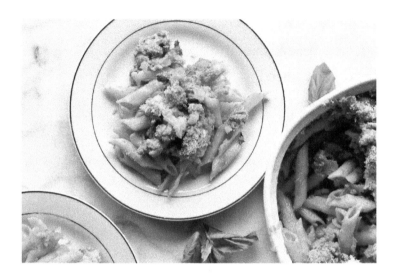

Prep:10 mins

Cook:20 mins

Easy

Serves 4

Ingredients
- 400g fusilli pasta
- 100g frozen pea
- 50g butter

- 50g plain flour
- 600ml milk
- 1 tsp Dijon mustard
- 2 x 195g cans tuna, drained
- 4 spring onions, sliced
- 198g can sweetcorn, drained
- 100g cheddar, grated

Directions:

1. Bring a pan of water to the boil. Add the pasta and cook, following pack instructions, until tender. Add the peas for the final 3 mins cooking time.

2. Meanwhile, melt the butter in a pan over a medium heat. Stir in the flour and cook for 2 mins. Add the milk, whisking constantly, then slowly bring to the boil, stirring often, until sauce thickens. Remove from the heat, add the mustard and season well.

3. Heat the grill to medium. Drain the pasta and peas, then return to the pan and stir in the tuna, spring onions, sweetcorn and sauce. Tip into a shallow baking dish, top with the cheddar and cook under the grill for 5 mins or until golden and bubbling.

Mulled apple juice

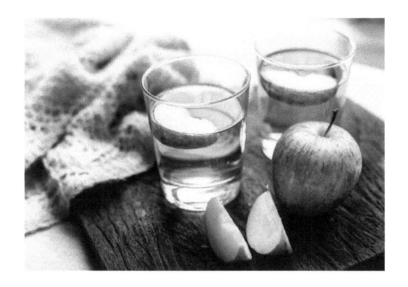

Prep: 5 mins

Cook: 10 mins

Easy

Serves 8

Ingredients

- 1l apple juice
- strips of orange peel
- 1 cinnamon stick, plus extra to garnish, if you like

- 3 cloves
- sugar or honey, to taste

Directions:

1. Simmer the apple juice with the strips of orange peel, cinnamon stick and cloves for about 5-10 mins until all the flavours have infused. Sweeten to taste

2. Serve each drink with a little orange peel and a piece of cinnamon stick, if you like.

Creamy linguine with ham, lemon & basil

Prep:10 mins

Cook:15 mins

Easy

Ingredients
• 400g linguine or spaghetti
• 90g pack prosciutto
• 1 tbsp olive oil
• juice 1 lemon
• 2 egg yolks
• 3 tbsp crème fraîche
• large handful basil leaves
• large handful grated parmesan, plus extra to serve, if you like

Directions:
1. Cook the linguine. Meanwhile, tear the ham into small pieces and fry in the olive oil until golden and crisp.

2. Drain the pasta, reserving a little of the cooking water, then return to the pan. Tip in the cooked ham. Mix together the lemon juice, egg yolks and crème fraîche, then add this to the pan along with the basil and

Parmesan. Mix in with tongs, adding a little of the cooking water, if needed, to make a creamy sauce that coats the pasta. Serve with extra Parmesan grated over the top, if you like.

Chicken nacho grills

Prep: 5 mins

Cook: 20 mins

Easy

Serves 4

Ingredients
- 40g bag tortilla chip
- 4 skinless chicken breasts
- 200g tub spicy tomato salsa
- 142ml pot soured cream
- handful grated mature cheddar

Directions:
1. Heat oven to 200C/fan 180C/gas 6. Crush the tortilla chips. Put the chicken breasts on a non-stick baking tray, season, then slash each 3 times with a knife. Spoon 1 tbsp of salsa on top of each, then 1 tbsp soured cream.
2. Sprinkle the chips over the chicken, then the cheese. Roast for 15-20 mins until the topping is golden and melting.

BBQ chicken with corn rice

Prep: 10 mins

Cook:40 mins

Easy

Serves 4

Ingredients

- 4 chicken leg portions, cut into thighs and drumsticks, skin removed
- 2 onions, 1 chopped, 1 cut into wedges
- 1 red and 1 green pepper, deseeded and thickly sliced
- 2 tbsp olive oil
- 200ml bottled barbecue sauce
- 2 tsp thyme leaves
- 250g long grain rice, rinsed
- 600ml chicken stock
- 340g can sweetcorn, rinsed and drained
- ½ red chilli, finely chopped (optional)

Directions:

1. Heat oven to 200C/180C fan/gas 6. Slash each piece of chicken 2-3 times. Put the chicken, onion wedges and peppers in a roasting tin or ovenproof pan, then toss with 1 tbsp oil and the barbecue sauce. Roast for 40 mins, turning halfway, until sticky and tender. Add a splash of water if the sauce dries up a little at the edges.

2. Meanwhile, heat 1 tbsp oil in a medium pan, then soften the chopped onion for 5 mins. Stir in the thyme, rice, stock and seasoning. Bring to the boil, cover and simmer for 12 mins. Turn off the heat, tip in the corn, add chilli if using, put the lid back on and let the rice steam for 10 mins more. Fluff up the rice, then serve with the chicken, vegetables and pan juices.

Mini elf doughnuts

Prep: 45 mins

Cook: 8 mins - 10 mins plus cooling

More effort

Makes 24

Ingredients
- 2 tbsp melted butter, plus an extra 1 tbsp for greasing
- 100g plain flour
- ½ tsp baking powder
- 1 tsp ground cinnamon
- ¼ tsp ground nutmeg
- 3 tbsp golden caster sugar
- 1 large egg
- 1 tsp vanilla extract
- 2 tbsp maple syrup
- 4 tbsp buttermilk For the icing
- 250g icing sugar
- 50ml milk
- red and green food colouring
- red, green & white sprinkles

• red and green writing icing tubes (optional)

Directions:

1. Heat oven to 180C/160C fan/gas 4. Brush some melted butter in the holes of a 24-hole mini muffin tin.

2. Put the flour, baking powder, cinnamon, nutmeg and sugar in a big bowl and mix together with your hands.

3. Pour the melted butter into a jug with the egg, vanilla, maple syrup and buttermilk, and mix together with a fork.

4. Pour the wet Ingredients over the dry ones and use a big wooden spoon to mix until there are no lumps.

5. Use teaspoons to divide the mixture between the holes in the tin. Bake in the oven for 8-10 mins, then cool in the tin.

6. Now it's time to turn them into doughnuts. Once cool, carefully tip the cakes out. Sit each on a chopping board and push an apple corer into the centre to cut the middle out so you have a ring.

7. Put the icing sugar and milk in a saucepan over a low heat. Whisk until runny and smooth. Divide the icing between three bowls, and mix a little green food colouring into one bowl, and a little red colouring into another.

8. Sit the doughnuts on a wire rack (so the drips can fall off), then spoon a little icing onto each. Decorate with sprinkles and writing icing, if you like. As this glaze dries quickly, finish decorating one colour, then start the next colour. If the icing is not runny enough, put in the microwave for 10 secs and stir well. Will keep for 2 days.

Chocolate-chip cookie ice-cream sandwiches

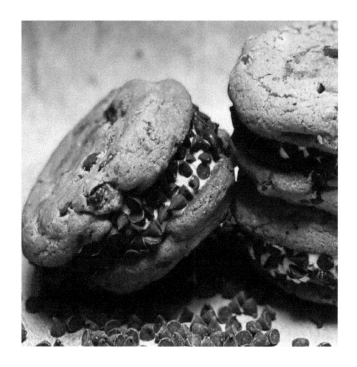

Prep:20 mins

Cook:20 mins Plus overnight chilling

Easy

Makes 12 sandwiches or 24 cookies

Ingredients

- 280g light soft brown sugar
- 225g granulated sugar
- 250g butter
- 2 large eggs
- 1 tbsp vanilla extract
- 450g plain flour
- 2 tsp baking powder
- 300g good-quality milk chocolate, roughly chopped into chunks
- vanilla ice cream, to serve

Directions:

1. To make the cookies, tip the sugars and butter into a large bowl. Get a grown-up to help you use an electric hand mixer to blend them together until the mixture looks smooth and creamy, and a little paler in colour.

2. Carefully break in the eggs, one at a time, mixing well between each egg and pausing to scrape down the sides with a spatula.

3. Mix in the vanilla. (To avoid unwanted crunchy bits, get your helper to crack the eggs into a separate bowl first, then it's easy to pick out any shell before tipping into the mixture.)

4. Sift in the flour and baking powder, then mix well with a wooden spoon.Stir through the chocolate chunks. Use your hands to squeeze the dough together in 1 big lump, then split into 2 even pieces. Put each piece on a sheet of cling film.

5. Roll each piece of dough in the cling film so that they form thick sausage shapes, then seal the ends. Put them in the fridge and chill for at least 3 hrs or overnight – can be frozen at this point. 6Heat oven to 180C/160C fan/ gas

6. Take the dough rolls out of the fridge, unwrap and use a small knife to slice each one into 12 pieces, so you have 24 in total.

7. Place the slices on a baking tray lined with baking parchment. Ask a grown-up to put this in the oven to bake for 20 mins or until the cookies are golden brown on the edges, but still pale in the centre.

8. Allow to cool slightly before lifting them onto a wire rack to cool completely. Sandwich the cookies together with ice cream and dig in!

Chicken pesto wrap

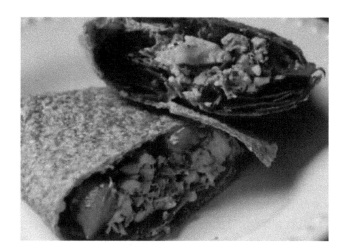

Prep:10 mins

No cook

Easy

Serves 2

Ingredients

- 1 cooked chicken breast, shredded
- 2 tbsp soured cream, plain yogurt or mayo
- 2 tsp pesto
- 2 thin slices mild cheese, such as Edam

- 2 flour tortillas
- handful chopped red pepper or sweetcorn kernels
- lettuce leaves

Directions:

1. Mix together the shredded chicken, soured cream, yogurt or mayonnaise with the pesto. Season.

2. Lay a slice of cheese on each wrap, then divide the chicken mixture between them. Sprinkle with red pepper or sweetcorn, then top with the lettuce leaves. Be careful not to overfill or it will be tricky to contain all the filling. Wrap and roll each one, then pack in a lunchbox or tightly wrap in foil.

Gooey brownies

Prep:10 mins

Cook:35 mins

Easy

Makes 16-20

Ingredients

• 100g unsalted butter, softened

• 175g caster sugar
• 2 large eggs, beaten
• 75g plain flour
• 50g cocoa powder
• 1 tsp baking powder
• 3 tbsp milk
• 4 tbsp mixed white and milk chocolate chips
• 100g milk chocolate
• 75g full-fat soft cheese

Directions:

1 Heat oven to 180C/160C fan/gas 4 and line a 20cm square brownie tin with baking parchment. Beat the butter and sugar together with an electric whisk, then add the eggs one by one. 2 Sift in the flour, cocoa powder and baking powder, and add the

milk. Mix everything together, then stir in the chocolate chips. Spoon into the tin and level the top. Bake for 30 mins, or until the top is set, then cool completely. 3Meanwhile, make the topping, melt the milk chocolate, cool a little, then mix it with the soft cheese until fully combined and silky.Spread the topping over the cooled brownies and cut into small squares – these are very rich.

Christmas cake cupcakes

Prep:40 mins

Cook:45 mins

Easy

Makes 12

Ingredients

For the batter
- 200g dark muscovado sugar
- 175g butter, chopped
- 700g luxury mixed dried fruit
- 50g glacé cherries
- 2 tsp grated fresh root ginger
- zest and juice 1 orange
- 100ml dark rum, brandy or orange juice
- 85g/3oz pecan nuts, roughly chopped
- 3large eggs, beaten
- 85g ground almond
- 200g plain flour
- ½ tsp baking powder
- 1 tsp mixed spice
- 1 tsp cinnamon For the icing
- 400g pack ready-rolled marzipan (we used Dr Oetker)
- 4 tbsp warm apricot jam or shredless marmalade
- 500g pack fondant icing sugar

- icing sugar, for dusting You will also need
- 6 gold and 6 silver muffin cases
- 6 gold and 6 silver sugared almonds
- snowflake sprinkles

Directions:

1. Tip the sugar, butter, dried fruit, whole cherries, ginger, orange zest and juice into a large pan. Pour over the rum, brandy or juice, then put on the heat and slowly bring to the boil, stirring frequently to melt the butter. Reduce the heat and bubble gently, uncovered for 10 mins, stirring every now and again to make sure the mixture doesn't catch on the bottom of the pan. Set aside for 30 mins to cool.

2. Stir the nuts, eggs and ground almonds into the fruit, then sift in the flour, baking powder and spices. Stir everything together gently but thoroughly. Your batter is ready.

3. Heat oven to 150C/130C fan/gas 2. Scoop the cake mix into 12 deep muffin cases (an ice-cream scoop works well), then level tops with a spoon dipped in hot water. Bake for 35-45 mins until golden and just firm to touch. A skewer inserted should come out clean. Cool on a wire rack.

4. Unravel the marzipan onto a work surface lightly dusted with icing sugar. Stamp out 12 rounds, 6cm across. Brush the cake tops with apricot jam, top with a marzipan round and press down lightly.

5. Make up the fondant icing to a spreading consistency, then swirl on top of each cupcake. Decorate with sugared almonds and snowflakes, then leave to set. Will keep in a tin for 3 weeks.

Fruity ice-lolly pens

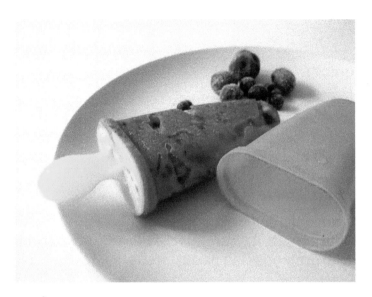

Prep:10 mins

Cook:15 mins - 20 mins

Easy

Makes 6

Ingredients
• 50ml sugar-free blackcurrant cordial
• 50ml sugar-free orange cordial
• 5 tsp each red and orange natural food colouring, plus extra for painting
• 50g blueberry

- 50g strawberry, chopped
- a few red grapes, halved

Directions:

1. Pour each cordial into a separate jug, and add the corresponding food colouring. Stir in 100ml water. Put the blueberries, strawberries and grapes into the ice-lolly moulds and pour the blackcurrant mixture up to the brim of 3 moulds. Pour the orange cordial into the remaining 3 moulds. Freeze for 4 hrs.

2. Remove the lollies from the moulds and dot extra food colouring onto a dish. Dip the lollies into the colouring and use to draw on clean paper– while enjoying the lolly at the same time.

Chocolate & raspberry pots

Prep: 15 mins

Cook: 10 mins

Serves 6

Ingredients

- 200g plain chocolate (not too bitter, 50% or less)
- 100g frozen raspberry, defrosted or fresh raspberries
- 500g Greek yogurt
- 3 tbsp honey
- chocolate curls or sprinkles, for serving

Directions:

1. Break the chocolate into small pieces and place in a heatproof bowl. Bring a little water to the boil in a small saucepan, then place the bowl of chocolate on top, making sure the bottom of the bowl does not touch the water. Leave the chocolate to melt slowly over a low heat.

2. Remove the chocolate from the heat and leave to cool for 10 mins. Meanwhile, divide the raspberries between 6 small ramekins or glasses.

3. When the chocolate has cooled slightly, quickly mix in the yogurt and honey. Spoon the chocolate mixture over the raspberries. Place in the fridge to cool, then finish the pots with a few chocolate shavings before serving.

89

Veggie noodle pot

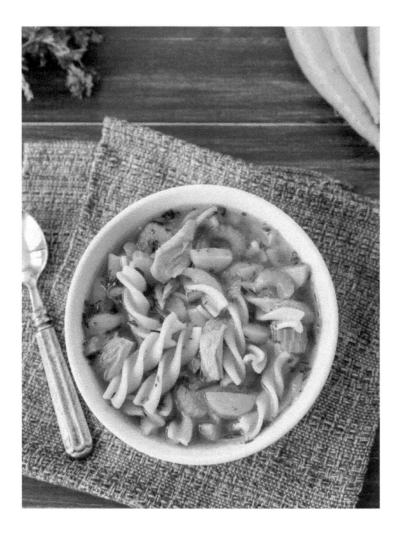

Prep: 10 mins

Cook: 10 mins

Easy

Serves 2

Ingredients

- 100g noodles (rice, soba or egg)
- 3 tbsp frozen peas
- handful sugar snap peas or mangetout, halved lengthways
- handful baby corn, halved lengthways
- 1 spring onion, sliced
- ½ red pepper, deseeded and chopped

For the dressing
- 1 tbsp reduced-salt soy sauce
- 1 tsp clear honey
- ½ garlic clove, crushed
- juice 1/2 lemon
- grating of fresh ginger (optional)

For the omelette
- 1 tbsp olive oil
- splash of milk
- 2 eggs, beaten

Directions:

1. To make the omelette, heat the olive oil in a small non-stick frying pan. Add a splash of milk to the beaten eggs, then tip into the pan. Stir once and allow to cook over a gentle heat until almost set. Flip (using a plate if necessary) and cook on the other side until cooked through. Tip onto a board and cut into strips. (You can roll

91

the omelette up and cut slices to give you spirals, if you like.)

2. Cook the noodles following pack instructions. Drain and rinse under cold water, then set aside. Meanwhile, mix the dressing Ingredients together. Blanch the peas and sugar snap peas, then drain and run under cold water to stop them cooking any further.

3. To assemble the salad, mix the noodles with the baby corn, spring onion, red pepper and green veg, then toss with the dressing and top with strips of omelette.

Mango crunch cookies

Prep: 15 mins

Cook:15 mins plus chilling and cooling

Easy

Makes about 14 large or 28 small cookies

Ingredients

• 140g butter, at room temperature
• 50g golden caster sugar
• 1 egg yolk
• 1 tsp vanilla extract
• 1 tbsp maple syrup
• 100g dried mango, roughly chopped
• 175g plain flour, plus extra for dusting To decorate (optional)
• 200g icing sugar, sifted
• 3 tbsp mango juice
• sprinkles

.Directions:.

1. Heat the oven to 180C/160C fan/gas 4. Place the butter
   and sugar in a food processor and blitz until smooth and
   creamy. Add the egg yolk, vanilla, maple syrup and mango.
   Whizz to blend in and chop the mango a little more finely.
   Add the flour and briefly blitz to form a soft dough. Turn

out onto a floured surface and shape into a ball. Chill for 20 mins.

2. Using a rolling pin, roll the cookie dough to the thickness of a £1 coin on a lightly floured surface, then cut out biscuit shapes with a 10cm cutter for large, or a 5cm cutter for smaller cookies.

3. Transfer to a baking tray lined with baking parchment, and cook for 12-15 mins or until lightly golden and firm. Remove and leave to cool on a wire rack.

4. If decorating, mix the icing sugar with the mango juice to make a runny icing. Drizzle or spoon the icing over the biscuits, then add the sprinkles if using, and leave to set. Will keep in a biscuit tin for up to 1 week.

Vegan gingerbread

Prep: 20 mins

Cook: 12 mins plus chilling

Easy

Serves 10

Ingredients

- 1tbsp ground flaxseed
- 140g dairy-free margarine
- 100g dark muscovado sugar
- 3tbsp golden syrup
- 350g plain flour, plus extra for dusting
- 1tsp bicarbonate of soda
- 1tbsp ground ginger
- 2tsp ground cinnamon

Directions:

1. Combine the flaxseed with 2½ tbsp water, and leave to thicken for 5 mins. Line two baking sheets with baking parchment. Melt the margarine, sugar and syrup in a pan over a low heat, then transfer to a medium bowl and leave to cool slightly. Stir in the flaxseed mix, then the flour,

bicarb, spices and a pinch of salt until it comes together into a smooth dough. Chill for 30-45 mins until firm.

2. Heat the oven to 200C/180C fan/gas 6. Roll the dough out on a lightly floured surface to a 5mm thickness. Stamp out as many gingerbread people as you can, then re-roll the trimmings and continue until all the dough is used. Put on the sheets and bake for 12 mins until golden. Leave to cool on the sheets for 10 mins, then transfer to wire racks to cool completely. Will keep in an airtight container for two weeks.

Cheese & ham pancake roll-ups

Prep:40 mins

Cook:50 mins

Easy

Serves a family of 4 (makes 8 pancakes)

Ingredients

For the pancakes
• 140g plain flour
• 2 eggs
• 25g butter, melted plus extra for buttering
• 350ml semi-skimmed milk
• sunflower or vegetable oil, for frying

For the roll-ups
• 12 thin slices of ham (125g pack), torn
• 260g bag spinach, cooked - see tip, below
• 140g grated cheddar
• 100ml half-fat crème fraîche
• 3 spring onions, sliced (optional)
• handful dried breadcrumbs

Directions:

1. <u>KIDS</u> the writing in bold is for you <u>ADULTS</u> the rest is for you. <u>FOR THE PANCAKES</u> Tip in the flour, make a well, crack the eggs in dishes – whisk together. Tip the flour into a mixing bowl and make a well in the middle. Crack the eggs into separate dishes, remove any shell, and add to the flour. Tip in the butter, add a little milk and whisk until smooth.

2. Whisk in the rest of the milk. Whisk in the rest of the milk, in a steady stream, until you have a smooth batter that is similar to the consistency of double cream. Now carefully pour the batter into a jug.

3. Wipe the pan with oil and pour in the batter. Using kitchen paper, wipe the pan with a little oil. Place the pan on the stove and heat until hot. Remove from the heat and pour in enough batter to cover the base, swirling it around. Return to the heat for 3 mins until the underside is cooked.

4. Now flip the pancake. Take the pan off the heat and, using a spatula, loosen the pancake. Flip the pancake in the air (or simply turn it over with the spatula) and cook the other side. When cooked, put the pancake to one side, then repeat the procedure to cook 7 more pancakes. <u>FOR THE ROLL-UPS</u> Butter a baking dish, then scatter ham and cheese over pancakes.

5. Heat oven to 200C/180C fan/gas 6. Butter a large baking dish. Now lay a pancake in front of you and scatter over some ham, spinach and cheese (remembering to save 25g of the cheese).

6. Roll up the pancakes and put them into the dish. Carefully roll up the pancakes and put them into the buttered dish. Repeat with all the pancakes.

7. Make the topping. In a small bowl, mix together the crème fraîche with the remaining cheese and spring onions, if you like.

8. Spread the topping, then sprinkle over the breadcrumbs. Spread the topping over the pancakes, sprinkle with breadcrumbs and bake for about 30 mins until bubbling and golden. Serve with a salad or veg.

Little jam tarts

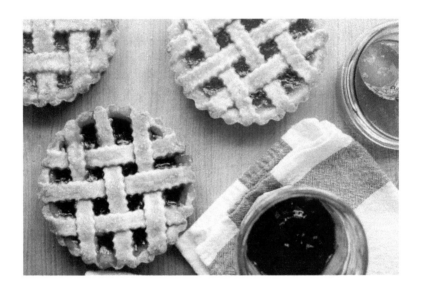

Prep:15 mins

Cook:15 mins

Easy

Makes 20

Ingredients
• 500g sweet shortcrust pastry
• 20 tsp jam (we used apricot, blackcurrant and strawberry)

Directions:

1. Roll out the shortcrust pastry on a lightly floured surface to just under the thickness of £1 coin. Stamp out 20 x 5cm circles using a pastry cutter and line 2 mini muffin tins (or make in 2 batches).

2. Prick with a fork and spoon 1 tsp jam into each (we used apricot, blackcurrant and strawberry). Stamp out shapes from the leftover pastry to decorate the tarts, if you like.

3. Bake at 200C/180C fan/gas 6 for 12-15 mins, until the pastry is golden.

Family meals: Easy fish cakes

Prep: 15 mins

Cook: 30 mins

Easy

Serves a family of 4-6 or makes 6-8 toddler meals

Ingredients
• 1 x pack fish pie mix (cod, salmon, smoked haddock etc, weight around 320g-400g depending on pack size)
• 3 spring onions, finely chopped
• 100ml milk
• 450g potato, peeled, large ones cut in half
• 75g frozen sweetcorn, defrosted
• handful of grated cheddar cheese
• 1 large egg, beaten
• flour, for dusting
• olive oil, for frying

Directions:

1. Cook the potatoes in boiling water until just tender. Drain well and return to the pan on a low heat. Heat for another minute or two to evaporate excess liquid. Mash the potato with a small knob of butter. Allow to cool.

2. Put the fish spring onions and milk in a shallow dish, cover with cling film and cook in the microwave for 1 ½ 2 mins until just cooked. If you don't have a microwave, put everything in a saucepan and gently cook until just opaque and cooked through.

3. Drain the fish and spring onions through a fine sieve. Gently mix through the potatoes, avoiding breaking up the fish too much, along with the sweetcorn, cheddar and a generous grind of black pepper. Form into 6 - 8 patties. The cooler the mash potato is when you do this, the easier it will be to form the patties as the mixture will be very soft when warm.

4. Pour the egg on one plate and scatter flour on the other. Dip the patties in egg and then flour and arrange on a sheet of baking paper on a tray. Put the patties in the fridge for at least half an hour to firm up if the patties feel very soft. At this point you can freeze the patties, wrapped individually. Defrost throughly before moving onto the next stage.

5. Heat a large frying pan with a generous glug of olive oil. When the oil is hot, carefully lower the fish cakes into the pan. Cook for 5 - 7 minutes or until golden brown underneath and then carefully flip them over. Fry for another 5 - 7 minutes or until golden on the bottom and heated all the way through.

Omelette wedges

Prep:20 mins

Cook:10 mins

Easy

Serves 6

Ingredients

- 3 spring onions
- 200g new potatoes
- 4 rashers smoked bacon
- 2 tbsp sunflower oil, plus 1 tsp
- 8 eggs
- 1 tsp English mustard (ready-made rather than powder)
- 85g mature cheddar
- 2 tomatoes

Directions:

1. Finely chop the spring onions and set aside. Thickly slice the potatoes (there is no need to peel them first), then boil in a pan of lightly salted water for 10 mins until just tender. Drain.

2. Meanwhile snip the bacon into pieces with scissors. Heat a frying pan with 1 tsp oil, then stir-fry the bacon until it

turns pink. Add the spring onions to the pan, stir briefly for a couple of secs to slightly soften, then tip the bacon and onion into a bowl. Wash and dry the frying pan.

3. Break the eggs into a bowl, then whisk with the mustard and a little salt and pepper. Make sure you don't get any shell into the mix. If you are worried you might, you can break the eggs into a cup, one at a time, before adding to the bowl – or ask an adult to break them for you.

4. Grate the cheese and add half to the egg mixture with the cooked bacon, onions and potatoes. Gently stir to mix everything. Heat 2 tbsp oil in the pan; when it is hot, pour in the mixture, then stir a couple of times as it sets on the base of the pan to start it cooking.

5. Turn on the grill so it has time to heat up. Leave the omelette to cook, undisturbed, over a low heat for about 6 mins. Meanwhile, cut the tomatoes into wedges, scatter over the omelette and sprinkle with the grated cheese.

6. When the omelette seems set on the base, but is still a little eggy on top, put the frying pan under the grill to cook the last of the egg mixture and melt the cheese. Cool for 5 mins, then turn out of the pan. Cut into wedges and serve with ketchup, toast, tea and orange juice for a delicious family breakfast.

Macadamia & cranberry American cookies

Prep: 20 mins

Cook: 12 mins

Easy

Makes 55

Ingredients
- 3 x 200g/7oz white chocolate bars, chopped
- 200g butter
- 2 eggs
- 100g light muscovado sugar
- 175g golden caster sugar
- 2 tsp vanilla extract
- 350g plain flour
- 2 tsp baking powder
- 1 tsp cinnamon
- 100g dried cranberry
- 100g macadamia nut, chopped

Directions:
1. Heat oven to 180C/160C fan/gas 4. Melt 170g of the chocolate, then allow to cool. Beat in the butter, eggs,

sugars and vanilla, preferably with an electric hand whisk, until creamy. Stir in the flour, baking powder, cinnamon and cranberries with two-thirds of the remaining chocolate and macadamias, to make a stiff dough.

2. Using a tablespoon measure or a small ice-cream scoop, drop small mounds onto a large baking dish, spacing them well apart, then poke in the reserved chocolate, nuts and berries. Bake in batches for 12 mins until pale golden, leave to harden for 1-2 mins, then cool on a wire rack.

3. To freeze, open-freeze the raw cookie dough scoops on baking trays; when solid, pack them into a freezer container, interleaving the layers with baking parchment. Use within 3 months. Bake from frozen for 15-20 mins.

Sweet snowballs

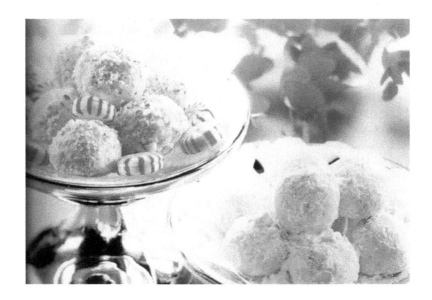

Prep: 20 mins

Cook: 5 mins Plus chilling

Easy

Makes 16

Ingredients

- 400g white chocolate, broken into pieces
- 100g rich tea biscuit
- 50g white Malteser

- 50g mini marshmallow
- 50g dried cranberries
- 50g cake crumbs (we used shop-bought Madeira cake)
- 3 tbsp golden syrup
- 100g desiccated coconut
- edible glitter (optional)

Directions:

1. Melt the chocolate in a bowl over a pan of simmering water. Meanwhile, crush the biscuits and Maltesers in a large bowl with a rolling pin.

2. Add mini marshmallows, dried cranberries and cake crumbs, then the chocolate and golden syrup. Mix well. Tip desiccated coconut onto a plate. Drop large spoonfuls of mixture onto the plate, then roll them around, coating in coconut and shaping into balls. Place on a baking tray and chill for 30 mins before serving. Sprinkle with edible glitter if you like.

Lightning Source UK Ltd.
Milton Keynes UK
UKHW020648120521
383579UK00001B/41